Page title

Information Regarding Breast Cancer

Table of contents

Introduction

The disease known as breast cancer is caused by abnormal breast cells that proliferate and develop into tumors. Tumors have the potential to grow throughout the body and become lethal if ignored. The milk ducts and/or the breast's milk-producing lobules are where breast cancer cells first proliferate. Breast cancer is a condition when the breast's cells proliferate uncontrollably. Breast cancer comes in various forms. Which breast cells develop into cancer determines the type of breast cancer. Most cases of breast cancer start in the lobules or ducts. Cancer cells have the ability to infiltrate adjacent healthy breast tissue and enter the lymph nodes under the arms, depending on the stage of breast cancer. Little organs called lymph nodes are responsible for removing foreign materials from the body. Cancer cells can spread to other areas of the body through the lymph fluid if they enter the lymph nodes.

Chapter 1

Breast cancer: what is it?

One of the most prevalent malignancies to strike women and those who identify as female at birth is breast cancer (AFAB). It happens when malignant cells in the breasts develop into tumors. An invasive breast cancer is one in which the tumor spreads to other parts of the body, accounting for about 80% of cases.

Although it usually affects women over 50, breast cancer can also strike women and people with AFAB under 50. Breast cancer is also a possibility for men and those who were designated male at birth (AMAB).

kinds of breast cancer

In order to customize treatment to be as effective as possible with the fewest possible side effects, healthcare experts identify the many types and subtypes of cancer. Typical forms of breast cancer consist of:

Milk ducts are the initial site of invasive (infiltrating) ductal carcinoma (IDC), a malignancy that spreads to neighboring breast tissue. In the US, this is the most prevalent kind of breast cancer.

Breast cancer that begins in the lobules, or milk-producing glands, of the breast frequently spreads to neighboring breast tissue. In the US, it is the second-most prevalent type of breast cancer.

Similar to IDC, ductal carcinoma in situ (DCIS) is a type of breast cancer that begins in the milk ducts. The distinction is that DCIS stays inside your milk ducts. Less frequent forms of breast cancer consist of: Triple-negative breast cancer (TNBC): Compared to other breast cancers, this invasive malignancy is more aggressive and spreads more quickly.

IBC, or inflammatory breast cancer, is an uncommon but rapidly spreading malignancy that resembles a rash on the breast. In the US, IBC is not common.

Breast illness caused by Paget's: This uncommon malignancy may appear as a rash that affects the skin around your nipple. Paget's disease of the breast accounts for less than 4% of all cases of breast cancer.

Subtypes of breast cancer

Breast cancer subtypes are categorized by the status of receptor cells by medical professionals. Protein particles on or on the surface of cells are known as receptors.

Certain molecules in your blood, such as hormones like progesterone and estrogen, can be drawn to or attached to them. Progesterone and estrogen promote the growth of malignant cells. Healthcare professionals can better plan the treatment of breast cancer by knowing whether the malignant cells contain progesterone or estrogen receptors.

ER-positive (ER+) breast tumors have estrogen

receptors, which is one of the subtypes.

Breast tumors that are PR-positive (PR+) have progesterone receptors.

Progesterone and estrogen receptors are found in breast tumors that are HR-positive (HR+).

Breast tumors classified as HR-negative (HR-) lack progesterone or estrogen receptors.

breast tumors that are HER2-positive (HER2+), meaning that their HER2 protein levels are higher than usual. This protein promotes the growth of cancer cells. A percentage of 15–20% of breast cancer cases are HER2-positive.

Statistics and facts about breast cancer

About 30% of all new instances of cancer among American women are diagnosed with breast cancer each year. Here are the most recent statistics and facts about breast cancer:.

Incidence rates of breast cancer started to decline in the US in 2000, following two decades of rising rates. Just from 2002 to 2003, they fell by 7%. According to one explanation, this decline was partly caused by women using hormone replacement therapy (HRT) less after the Women's Health Initiative study's findings were released in 2002. These findings pointed to a link between a higher risk of breast cancer and hormone replacement therapy. The incidence rates have gone up by 0.5% annually in recent years. Lung cancer is the primary cause of cancer-related mortality among American women, with breast cancer coming in second.

What is the frequency of breast cancer?

Breast cancer is the most frequent cancer globally, accounting for 12.5% of all new cases reported each year.

The most prevalent malignancy among American women's diagnoses is breast cancer. Breast cancer accounts for almost 30% of all newly diagnosed malignancies in women each year.

One in eight American women, or almost 13% of all women, will eventually get invasive breast cancer.

It is anticipated that 297,790 new instances of invasive

breast cancer and 55,720 new cases of DCIS will be detected in American women in 2023. An estimated 2,800 men will receive a diagnosis of invasive breast cancer in 2023. The lifetime risk of breast cancer for men is approximately 1 in 833. In the United States, there are currently over four million women who have experienced breast cancer. This applies to ladies who have completed their treatment as well as those who are undergoing it. Less than 1% of breast cancer cases in the US are diagnosed in men. Facts about breast cancer age at diagnosis Half of women with breast cancer receive a diagnosis before the age of 62, while the other half receive a diagnosis after.

This indicates that the median age at the time of breast cancer diagnosis is 62. Only approximately one in eight invasive breast cancers is detected in women under 45, whereas about two out of every three invasive breast cancers are found in women 55 and older. Breast cancer diagnoses are thus comparatively uncommon in younger women. Risk of breast cancer These are just a handful of the many breast cancer risk factors to be aware of.

From birth until old age, sexuality The two biggest risk factors for breast cancer are aging and being a woman. It's critical that you discuss your individual risk level with your doctor if you identify as transgender or nonbinary so that you may schedule screenings as frequently as is practical for you.

Family background If a woman has a first-degree family member (such as a mother, sister, or daughter) who has been diagnosed with breast cancer, her risk of developing the disease almost doubles. 15% of breast cancer patients report having a family member with the disease. Molecular Biology It is estimated that known gene mutations inherited from one's father or mother account for 5% to 10% of breast cancer cases. The most frequent mutations are found in the BRCA1 and BRCA2 genes.

Women without a family history of breast cancer

account for about 85% of cases of breast cancer. Rather than being inherited, these are caused by genetic mutations that arise from aging and life in general.

Women who carry a BRCA1 mutation have a lifetime risk of up to 72% of breast cancer. A BRCA2 mutation can put women at risk of up to 69%. Breast cancer in younger women is more likely to develop if they test positive for either the BRCA1 or BRCA2 mutation. These genetic alterations also come with an elevated risk of ovarian cancer. BRCA1 mutations are a less common cause of breast cancer in men, whereas BRCA2 mutations carry a lifetime risk of approximately 6.8%.

Racial and ethnic inequalities in breast cancer

The incidence and death rates of breast cancer continue to differ. Compared to women of other races or ethnicities, black women have a higher risk of dying from breast cancer.

Experts surmise that part of the reason for this is that, more than any other racial or ethnic group, black women are diagnosed with triple-negative breast cancer more often than any other. For black and Latina women in the US, breast cancer is the primary cause of cancer-related death. In the United States, breast cancer ranks second in terms of cancer-related deaths, after lung cancer, among women who are Asian and Pacific Islander, American Indian and Alaska Native, and white. Women of Ashkenazi Jewish descent are more likely to carry BRCA mutations, which increases their risk of breast cancer.

Chapter 2

Breast Cancer Stages

Your doctor will inform you of the stage of your cancer at the time of diagnosis. That will give an idea of the cancer's size and extent of dissemination. Stages I through IV are commonly used to categorize cancer, with IV being the most severe. These broad categories are derived from a much more intricate system that includes particulars about the tumor and its effects on the body as a whole. Knowing your cancer stage is crucial for a number of reasons, including:

Therapy: It aids your doctor in determining the most effective course of action. While chemotherapy may be necessary for an advanced-stage cancer, surgery may be necessary for an early-stage cancer.

Prospects: The time of cancer detection will have an impact on how quickly you recover. You can see what results are conceivable for you based on your stage.

Research: The majority of hospitals employ a nationwide database to monitor the therapies administered and their efficacy. To identify the best treatments, researchers can compare cases that are similar to each other.

Groups for Staging

To determine your overall stage, your doctor may utilize data from the tumor itself (pathologic stage) or from test results (clinical stage). The majority of tumor-involving malignancies are classified into five major categories. Typically, these are denoted by Roman numerals. Other types have their own staging methods, such as lymphomas, brain tumors, and blood cancers. However, they all disclose the cancer's stage of progression.

Stage 0 denotes the absence of cancer and the presence of aberrant cells that may develop into cancer. Another name for this is cancer in situ. Stage I denotes a localized, small-scale malignancy. Another name for this is early-stage cancer. Stages II and III indicate an advanced stage of the malignancy that has spread to neighboring tissues or lymph nodes.

When a cancer is in stage IV, it has spread to other bodily areas. Another name for it is metastatic, or advanced cancer.

Your clinical stage, or the approximate extent of the cancer's spread, is determined by a physical examination and a number of tests. Blood tests, further lab tests, and imaging scans are examples of tests. X-rays or any of the following could be those.

MRIs, or magnetic resonance imaging, use radio waves and strong magnets to create finely detailed photographs of the affected area.

Computerized tomography (CT) scan: Multiple X-rays

are combined to provide additional information by taking them from various angles. Ultrasound: Images of the interior of your body are created using high-frequency sound waves. Another option is a biopsy, which entails taking a small sample of tissue and examining it under a microscope. Your doctor will get additional information about the tumor and its effects on your body if it is surgically removed. Your test results are combined with that information to determine the pathologic stage, also known as the surgical stage. This is seen to be more accurate than the clinical stage, and it may **differ from it.**

TNM   Framework
Your doctor will also likely use the TNM system—an acronym for tumor, node, and metastasis—to assess the overall stage of your cancer. Each of these will be measured, and if a measurement cannot be made, it will be assigned a number or an "X.". Although the symbols for each type of cancer vary slightly, they generally

mean the same thing:

Tumor (T): The letter "T" followed by a number between 0 and 4 indicates the size of the tumor and, in certain cases, its location. T0 denotes the absence of any detectable tumor. The tumor size increases with increasing numbers.

Node (N): If your lymph nodes have been affected by cancer, the number 0–3 after "N" indicates this. These glands have the function of filtering bacteria and viruses before they can spread to other parts of your body. N0 denotes the absence of lymph nodes. A larger number suggests the cancer is in more lymph nodes, farther distant from the initial tumor. Metastasis (M): "M" is followed by either 0 or 1. It says if the cancer has escalated to organs and tissues in other parts of the body. A 0 signifies it hasn't, while a 1 means it has.

Other **Factors**

Doctors Look at other facts about your cancer for signs

about how it will behave. These include:

Category: This is how cancer cells appear under a microscope. Low class indicates they look a lot like normal cells. A high grade indicates they look really weird. Low-class cancer cells develop more slowly and are less likely to escalate than high-grade cancer cells

.

Location: Where the tumor is in your body may make it tougher to treat.

Tumor markers: These are things in your blood or urine that are at higher levels when you have specific kinds of cancer.

Genetics: The cancer cells' DNA can inform your physician about the likelihood of metastasis and potential treatment options.

Your doctor can establish your total stage once they have all this information and have given you T, N, and M values.

The stages don't change. Your cancer stage often stays the same from the time of initial diagnosis, regardless of the course of the disease. For example, if your lung cancer is diagnosed at stage II, it will remain at that stage even if it goes into remission or spreads. The cancer cells vanish at that stage. This is because you have more treatment options and recovery chances the earlier your cancer is detected. Rediagnosis of some cancers is possible with further tests following treatment or if the cancer returns.

Chapter 3

Indications and Sources

Common signs of breast cancer and how to spot them.

What signs and symptoms accompany breast cancer? The disease may have a variety of effects on your breasts. Breast cancer symptoms might be easily recognized in certain cases. Some may just seem like different parts of your breast than the others. Furthermore, breast cancer may not exhibit any symptoms at all. However, if it does, some possible signs are   as   follows: changes to the shape, size, or profile of your breasts. a cluster or lump that resembles a pea in substance. a lump or thickening under your arms or in your breast area that persists throughout the menstrual cycle. a change in the appearance or feel of the skin around your breasts or nipples. There could be scaliness, puckering, dimples, or irritation on the skin. In comparison to other parts of your breast, it may appear darker,   redder,   or   purple. a firm, marble-like region under your skin. a fluid flow from your nipple that is clear or bloodstained.

Why   does   breast   cancer   develop? Experts know that breast cancer arises because breast cells have the ability to change into malignant cells that multiply and grow to form tumors. They are unsure about the cause of the change. However, the study's findings suggest that a lot of risk factors may increase your chance of developing breast cancer. 55 years of age or older is one of them.

Sex: People, especially women_AFAB individuals, have a considerably higher likelihood of having AMAB than do men or those without the disease.

Family background: If any of your parents, siblings, kids, or other close relatives currently have breast cancer, then you have an increased risk of developing the disease yourself.

Genetics: Up to 15% of breast cancer cases are caused by hereditary genetic changes. The most often mutated genes are BRCA1 and BRCA2.

Smoking: A number of malignancies, including breast cancer, have been linked to the use of tobacco products. Drinking beverages containing **alcohol:** Research indicates that drinking beverages containing alcohol may increase the risk of breast cancer. having a weight problem.

Radiation exposure: If you have ever undergone radiation therapy, especially to the head, neck, or chest, your chance of developing breast cancer is enhanced. **Hormone replacement therapy:** The likelihood of receiving a diagnosis of the condition is higher for those who use hormone replacement therapy (HRT).

What adverse effects could breast cancer bring on? The most dangerous side effect is metastatic breast cancer, which is breast cancer that spreads to other regions of the body, such as the brain, bones, liver, and lungs. According to the study, nearly one in three women and AFAB individuals with early-stage disease go on to develop metastatic breast cancer.

How is breast cancer detected?

Medical experts may order mammograms or conduct physical examinations to look for signs of breast cancer. However, they perform the following tests to determine the illness: mammography using ultrasound. breast magnetic resonance imaging (MRI) scan. MRI of the breast. immunohistochemical identification of hormone receptors.

genetic tests to identify the breast cancer-causing mutations.

Breast cancer stages Systems for staging cancer are used by medical professionals to plan patient care. Providers can better determine a patient's prognosis—what to expect following treatment—by staging the malignancy.

The staging of breast cancer is determined by the kind of breast cancer, the location and size of the tumor, and if the cancer has spread to other parts of the body. The stages of breast cancer are:
Stage 0: Your breast ducts are the only areas of your breast where the disease has not spread, indicating that it is noninvasive.
Stage I: Neighboring breast tissue contains malignant cells.
Stage II: A tumor or tumors have been produced by the malignant cells. The tumor can be greater than 5 centimeters wide but not larger than 2 centimeters across, or it can be smaller than 2 centimeters across and have migrated to lymph nodes under the arms. At this stage, tumors can range in size from 2 to 5 cm in diameter and may or may not impact the lymph nodes in the surrounding area.
Stage III: surrounding tissues and lymph nodes have breast cancer.
Stage IV: Your breast cancer has progressed to other

parts of your body, such as your bones, liver, lungs, or brain.

Treatments of breast cancer

The major treatment for breast cancer is surgery, though medical professionals may employ other methods as well. One type of surgery for breast cancer is a mastectomy. Lump removal and reconstruction of the breast. Surgical procedures can be combined by providers with one or more of the following therapies: chemotherapy and radiation treatment, which includes radiation administered during surgery (IORT). immunotherapy, which includes treatment with selective estrogen receptor modulators (SERMs). focused treatment. What adverse effects are associated with treatment? Weakness, nausea, and vomiting are typical side effects of radiation and chemotherapy. Similar side effects to immunotherapy, hormone treatment, and targeted therapy include gastrointestinal problems such as diarrhea and constipation. Individuals respond to breast cancer therapy in different ways. Ask your healthcare practitioner about the potential side effects of your therapy, including how they might impact your day-to-day activities, if you are undergoing it. Consult your physician about palliative care as well. In order to make your treatment experience as comfortable as possible, palliative care assists in managing the symptoms of breast cancer and the side effects of the medication. Surgical complications related to breast cancer Breast cancer surgery is not an exception to the rule that all procedures include some risk of complications. It's crucial to keep in mind that surgery can remove cancer that could be fatal while you weigh your options. The risks of breast cancer are generally greater than the complications.

Ask your medical professional to go over any possible side effects if you are having breast cancer surgery. These could include infection at the location of surgery. clots of blood that may form following surgery. harm to nerves. edema lymphatic

Chapter 4

Preventions of Breast Cancer

Is it possible to prevent breast cancer? It's possible that breast cancer cannot be prevented. However, you can lower your chance of getting it. Not to mention, routine mammograms and self-examinations can aid in the early detection of breast cancer when treatment options are more favorable.

How may my risk be reduced?

The American Cancer Society (ACS) offers the following guidance for all women, including those who are AFAB, while there is no sure-fire method to lower the risk of breast cancer: Reach and maintain a healthy weight—this is the weight that suits you best. Consult a medical professional for advice on establishing a healthy weight-management program.
Consume a balanced diet: According to certain research, eating a diet high in fruits, vegetables, dairy products, and lean protein can lower your risk of developing breast cancer

Steer clear of processed and red meat to lower your risk.
Get going: Regular physical activity reduces the risk of breast cancer, according to studies. Steer clear of alcoholic beverages. Research demonstrates a connection between alcohol and breast cancer. According to the American Medical Association, women and individuals who are AFAB should only have one drink each day. Obtain a screening When tumors are too tiny to feel, mammograms are frequently used to find them. Self-examination on a regular basis will help you detect

breast cancerous tumors and maintain the health of your breasts.

Due to genetic mutations they inherited or because family members had the disease, some women and people who identify as AFAB are more likely to get breast cancer. In that case, you might want to think about the following: searching for breast cancer genes genetically. medications such as aromatase inhibitors, raloxifene, and tamoxifen that may reduce the risk of breast cancer. mastectomy performed as a prophylactic measure. regular physical exams and testing for breast cancer.

Ask your doctor if you need to have any additional tests to identify breast cancer if you have an elevated risk of the disease, especially if you are under 40. **What is the breast cancer survivor rate?** Breast cancer survival rates differ depending on a number of variables, including the kind, stage, and invasion or noninvasiveness of the malignancy. The National Cancer Institute (US) maintained statistics that showed 91% of patients with breast cancer were still living five years following their diagnosis. The institute groups survival rates for breast cancer according to stages:

Local: There is no external cancer spreading from your breast.

Regional: Neighboring lymph nodes and tissue have been affected by cancer.

Distant: Cancer is found in more remote parts of the body, such as the lungs or liver. Recall that breast cancer survival numbers are simply approximations derived from the experiences of other people. Different people are affected by cancer in different ways. Speak with your healthcare professional if you have any specific questions about cancer survival rates. They are your best resource, as they are aware of your circumstances.

How good is the prognosis for breast cancer? As of right now, fewer people are losing their lives to breast cancer, and more people are receiving early-stage diagnoses, which makes the disease simpler to cure. Five years after their diagnosis, 99% of patients with early-stage breast cancer were still alive, according to the data. They might be thought to be free of breast cancer in some circumstances. Nevertheless, breast cancer can recur, and if it does, it might do so as metastatic breast cancer.

Race may also affect one's outlook. The American Cancer Society states that, compared to white women, black women and individuals with AFAB have a somewhat lower risk of breast cancer. However, compared to white women, black women had a higher breast cancer death rate.

Coexisting With breast cancer

How do I look after my needs?

It might not be easy to live with breast cancer. There may be days when everything seems too much for you. Think about the following advice for looking after yourself during the diagnosis and treatment of breast cancer:

Make time for rest. Treatment for breast cancer can be very draining. Remind yourself to take breaks when necessary, not just when you feel like you have the time. **Consume healthfully.** Your appetite may change as a result of treatment. You can maintain your strength during treatment by eating a diet rich in fruits, vegetables, lean protein, and whole grains. **Control your tension.** Stress is cancer. Engaging in regular walks or workout programs can be beneficial. Seek assistance: From the day of your diagnosis until now, you have been living with breast cancer. Inquire with your healthcare provider about cancer survivorship programs, as they may be able to assist you in coping with some of the difficulties associated with having breast cancer.

When should I visit my medical professional?

If you experience new symptoms, such as pain or weakness in a different body part, or if your symptoms seem to be getting worse, get in touch with your healthcare professional.

When is the best time for me to visit the ER? If your response to cancer therapy is more intense than you anticipated, you should visit the emergency room. For instance, if you're constantly vomiting and are seriously dehydrated, you should visit the emergency hospital.

What inquiries ought I make of my healthcare professional?

When most people first find out they have breast cancer, they have a lot of questions. The following are some potential inquiries you should make of your provider: Which kind of breast cancer am I experiencing? What is the size, grade, and stage of the tumor? What is the status of my progesterone and estrogen receptors?
What level of HER2 am I at? Will surgery be necessary for me? What additional choices are there for treatment? Do I have access to a clinical trial? Other Frequently Asked Questions How long may breast cancer go undiagnosed? It may take years for breast cancer symptoms to manifest, such as breast lumps. However, not every bulge or bump is malignant. If you have a strange lump or bump that doesn't go away after a few days, see a doctor.

At what pace does breast cancer progress?

That is dependent upon a number of variables, such as the kind of breast cancer you have, whether it is inherited, and the stage and grade of the tumor. Ask your healthcare practitioner about what to expect if you have been diagnosed with breast cancer. Is breast cancer a symptom specific to men? Breast cancer does occur in men and people with AMAB, but it is uncommon. Less than 1% of all occurrences of male breast cancer occur in the United States, where 2,600 men are affected annually. Compared to cisgender men, transgender women are more likely to get breast cancer. In addition, compared to cisgender women, transgender men had a lower risk of breast cancer.

Lifestyle Factors Increasing the Risk of Breast Cancer

Except for skin cancer, breast cancer is the most common cancer among women worldwide. One in eight women in the United States may receive a breast cancer diagnosis at some point in their lives. Cancers are complicated illnesses with a wide range of underlying causes. However, a few lifestyle choices may increase your risk of breast cancer. Being affected by one or more of these characteristics does not guarantee an illness. Furthermore, even in the absence of any risk factors, breast cancer can still develop.

Weight: Over 70% of adult Americans are overweight or obese. Gaining weight increases your chance of breast cancer, particularly if you do it after menopause. Furthermore, a higher chance of cancer recurrence is associated with obesity or being overweight. But not every fat is created equal. More harmful than the sort on your thighs or hips is the kind that surrounds your abdomen.

It produces the hormone insulin, which, if produced in excess, may encourage the spread of cancer cells.

Reducing your body weight by even 5%–10% can have an impact. If you're trying to lose weight, try to shed half a pound a week until you reach your target. booze.

Excessive alcohol use increases the levels of estrogen and other hormones associated with breast cancer. It might also harm the cells in your DNA. Your risk increases by 15% if you consume three or more alcoholic beverages per week. If you exceed three drinks per day, it increases by an additional 10%. Drinks without alcohol are a risk-free option. smoking. If you began smoking before the age of 17, your risk of developing breast cancer increased. Your risk will stay elevated for approximately 20 years after you stop. You can consult your doctor about medicine or a patch if you need assistance quitting. Join a support group for quitting smoking. Try meditation and acupuncture. hormones. Breast cancer rates among women who had completed menopause, or postmenopausal women, decreased in the early 2000s when many of them, at the suggestion of medical professionals, ceased using hormone replacement therapy (HRT).

Risk increases with progesterone and estrogen HRT administered at menopause for longer than five years. Similarly, birth control tablets might work. Hormones are released in trace amounts by them. There is less risk when you quit taking them.

What stage of breast cancer do we have?

hormones. Breast cancer rates among women who had completed menopause, or postmenopausal women, decreased in the early 2000s when many of them, at the suggestion of medical professionals, ceased using hormone replacement therapy (HRT). Risk increases with progesterone and estrogen HRT administered at menopause for longer than five years. Similarly, birth control tablets might work. Hormones are released in trace amounts by them. There is less risk when you quit taking them. radiation. We are surrounded by this electromagnetic wave energy, which comes from sources like X-rays used in medicine and the earth. Studies indicate that there might be a link between radiation and breast cancer. However, the relationship between radiofrequency radiation, a separate type of low-energy radiation that is emitted by Bluetooth, Wi-Fi, and cell phones, and cancer is not entirely established. postponed having children. In the United States, one in six new mothers is older than 35. If you become pregnant for the first time after turning 30, your chance of breast cancer increases. This is because, during the course of your lifetime, you get exposed to more estrogen. Most breast cancers grow because of estrogen. Additionally, pregnancy can shield you from cancer-causing abnormal cell development. Passivity. Modern life is largely spent sitting down. Sedentary lifestyles increase the risk of breast cancer and obesity. Seek out methods to keep moving. . Look for something to do to get off the couch. At least 150 minutes of moderately strenuous exercise per week, such as riding a bike or doing yoga, is recommended by the American Cancer Society. inadequate vitamin D. You may be more susceptible to breast cancer if your levels are low. Vitamin D is derived from several foods and supplements. When sunlight strikes your skin, your body produces it. It may potentially halt the spread of cancer.

Compared to people in warmer climates, breast cancer claims the lives of more people in the Northeastern United States. However, excessive sun exposure increases the risk of skin cancer. Generally, three times a week for fifteen minutes in the sun is sufficient. Poor diet. A diet abundant in highly processed foods, such as cookies, chips, and candies, and low in whole foods, such as whole grains and fresh produce, is considered unhealthy. This might increase your chance of cancer.

Consuming a lot of red and processed meats may also help. Chemicals that cause cancer are absorbed by food cooked to high temperatures. Limit your weekly intake of red meat to three portions. There are 12–18 ounces in all. According to a study, young women who consumed large amounts of red meat during their adolescent and early adult years were at a 22% increased risk of developing breast cancer in later life.

Changed Words

Structural Changes

Chapter 5

Food decisions that can help prevent breast cancer

Breast cancer cannot be prevented or caused by a single food or diet, but a person's dietary choices might influence their chance of getting the disease or their quality of life when it does.

Breast cancer is a complicated illness with numerous underlying causes. Age, gender, genetics, and family history are a few of these variables that are out of an individual's control.

On the other hand, there are some things that an individual can influence, like food, body weight, physical activity levels, and smoking. A small percentage of malignancies (30–40%) may be caused by dietary variables, according to some experts.

foods to consume

Breast cancer can develop in a variety of ways, start in unexpected locations, and require various treatments. Certain malignancies react better to certain foods, just as some cancer types respond better to certain treatments. In addition to contributing to a generally healthy diet, the following foods may help stop breast cancer from starting or spreading:

a range of fruits and veggies, including high-fiber salad items such as whole grains, beans, and lentils.

dairy and low-fat milk products

goods made from soybeans

meals high in other vitamins and vitamin D

foods with anti-inflammatory qualities, especially spices

foods high in antioxidants, primarily plant-based foods

Dietary regimens that give priority to these foods consist of:

a cuisine heavy in cooked greens, legumes, and sweet potatoes that is typical of the South

A Mediterranean diet that prioritizes wholesome oils and fresh fruits and vegetables

Any "prudent" diet rich in whole grains, seafood, fruit, and veggies

Vegetables and fruits

According to a study including 91,779 women, eating a diet high in plant-based foods could reduce the incidence of breast cancer by 15%. Fruits and vegetables are rich in flavonoids and carotenoids, which appear to offer a number of medical benefits in addition to their other advantages. The following foods may help prevent breast cancer, according to studies:

foliage, dark green veggies like broccoli and kale, and fruits, particularly berries and peaches

Fish, eggs, beans, lentils, and some meat

Naturally found in vegetables like carrots, beta-carotene has been linked by researchers to a lower risk of breast cancer. Researchers hypothesize that this could be the result of it interfering with cancer cells' ability to proliferate.

Between five and nine servings of fresh fruit and vegetables should be consumed each day, according to the United States Department of Agriculture (USDA). Fiber in the diet and antioxidants Although there is currently conflicting research on dietary fiber's relationship to breast cancer, a number of studies have suggested that it may offer some protection from the condition. Some forms of breast cancer may develop and spread more quickly as a result of excess estrogen. Preventing estrogen from interacting with breast cancer cells is the goal of certain therapies. Consuming a diet rich in fiber can help facilitate this process and hasten the removal of estrogen.

Fiber aids in the normal removal of waste, particularly excess estrogen, from the body and the digestive system. It lessens the harm that pollutants might cause and aids in the body's elimination. The way fiber binds to estrogen in the gastrointestinal tract might also aid in limiting the amount of estrogen the body absorbs. These elements might lower the chance of developing breast cancer. In addition to providing fiber, fruits, vegetables, whole grains, and legumes also have antioxidants, including beta-carotene and vitamins C and E. Because antioxidants lower the levels of free radicals—waste products that the body naturally produces—they can aid in the prevention of many diseases. A meta-analysis conducted in 2013 suggested that eating more whole grains could reduce the risk of breast cancer.

Healthy fat

Obesity is a condition that can be brought on by fatty meals, and those who are obese seem to be more susceptible to cancer, particularly breast cancer. The body needs some fat in food to function correctly, but the type of fat you eat matters. When consumed in moderation, monounsaturated and polyunsaturated fats can be advantageous. They can be found in: olive oil nuts, seeds, and avocados Fish from cold water, including salmon and herring, are high in omega-3 fat, which is a beneficial polyunsaturated lipid. Additionally, this fat might lower the risk of breast cancer. Find out more about good fats here. A 2015 study's authors referenced a rodent study in which they found that rats fed 8–25% omega-3 fats looked to have a 20–35% decreased risk of breast cancer. They also mentioned another study that included more than 3,000 women and revealed that those who ate a lot of omega-3 had a 25% decreased chance of developing breast cancer again in the next seven years. Omega-3 fatty acids may provide health benefits because of their anti-inflammatory properties. Breast cancer may have inflammation as a contributing component.

Soy

One nutritious food that may help lower the risk of breast cancer is soy. It is a plant-based product that is low in carbohydrates and high in protein, good fat, vitamins, and minerals. It also has isoflavones, which are antioxidants.

A 2017 study's authors examined data from 6,235 women and came to the general conclusion that "a higher dietary intake of isoflavone was associated with reduced all-cause mortality." The purpose of the study was to see if eating soy was beneficial for those who had breast cancer.

In addition to lowering heart disease risk, soy may also help lower levels of low-density lipoprotein (LDL), or "bad" cholesterol. These illnesses are risk factors for metabolic syndrome, which includes inflammation in addition to obesity. Although its exact significance in breast cancer is still unknown, inflammation may be involved. There is soy in meals like tempeh, edamame, and tofu. dairy substitute soybeans

Isoflavones, which are similar to estrogen, have led some individuals to wonder if soy could raise the risk of breast cancer.

But the author of a review paper from 2016 points out that isoflavones and estrogen are not the same thing, and they are not likely to act in the same manner. The North American Menopause Society has determined, according to the author, that isoflavones do not raise the risk of breast cancer.

foods to stay away from. Foods that could put you at risk Among the reliable sources of various cancers, including breast cancer, are fat, sugar, and added alcohol. Prepared meals and red meat

Research on alcohol has revealed a connection between frequent alcohol use and a higher risk of breast cancer. Alcohol may raise estrogen levels and harm DNA, according to breastcancer.org. Additionally, they point out that women who consume three alcoholic beverages each week have a 15% higher chance of getting breast cancer.

An extra drink a day increases the risk by approximately 10%, according to estimates.

Sweetener

According to a 2016 study, mice fed a diet as high in sugar as the average American diet had an increased risk of developing mammary gland tumors, which are identical to human breast cancer. Furthermore, there is a higher chance that these tumors will metastasize.

Research on fat indicates that not all fats are harmful. Certain plant-based lipids may help lower the risk of breast cancer, even while fat from processed foods seems to raise it. One kind of fat that is frequently found in prepared and processed meals is trans fat. Researchers have connected it to an increased risk of breast cancer. The majority of processed meals, including fried dishes, some crackers, donuts, and packaged cookies or pastries, contain trans fats. When possible, people should reduce the amount of trans fat they eat.

crimson meat

Red meat consumption has been linked in some studies to a higher risk of breast cancer, particularly if the meat is cooked to a high temperature, which can cause toxins to be released. Furthermore, cold cuts and processed meats frequently include high levels of fat, salt, and preservatives. These could make breast cancer more likely to occur rather than less. In general, foods that have undergone minimal preparation are healthier.

Additional advice

Sunlight exposure and diets high in vitamin D may help prevent breast cancer. Foods such as eggs, cold-water fish, and fortified foods all contain vitamin D. A person can get their vitamin D levels checked by seeing a doctor. If levels are low, a supplement might be suggested by the physician. There are a number of potential health benefits to green tea. The antioxidants included in it may support a stronger immune system and lower the incidence of breast cancer. The yellow spice known as turmeric may have anti-inflammatory qualities that slow the spread of breast cancer cells.

In general, maintaining a healthy body weight is good for wellbeing, but it's especially crucial for those who want to stop breast cancer from developing or coming back. One established risk factor for the illness is obesity.

It's also necessary to exercise. According to the National Cancer Institute, women who engage in at least four hours of weekly exercise are less likely to develop breast cancer.

It may be helpful to speak with other individuals who have the illness, trade recipes, and share experiences about which meals have been helpful

Chapter 6

Breast cancer with metastases

Cancer that has spread from your breast to other parts of your body is known as metastatic breast cancer, also known as advanced breast cancer or Stage IV breast cancer. Although there isn't a cure, more people with metastatic breast cancer are living longer than ever before because of improved therapies. **What is the breast cancer that has spread?** Breast cancer that has spread (metastasized) from your breast to other parts of your body is known as metastatic breast cancer, advanced breast cancer, or stage IV breast cancer. Although medical professionals are unable to treat metastatic breast cancer, they can suggest therapies that will prolong your life and enhance your quality of life. In actuality, as medical professionals discover novel approaches to treating metastatic breast cancer, more patients are experiencing longer survival times.

Is breast cancer with metastases common? According to the most recent data available, around 170,000 American women and individuals classified as female at birth (AFAB) are coping with metastatic breast cancer. According to predictions from the National Cancer Institute (NCI) in the United States, 2,800 men and individuals assigned male at birth (AMAB) and 297,000 women and people assigned AFAB will be diagnosed with breast cancer in 2023. Does breast cancer develop in everyone who has it? No, they don't. About 20% to 30% of women and persons with AFAB with early-stage disease go on to develop metastatic breast cancer, according to NCI data.

Signs and Origins

What are the signs of breast cancer that have spread? You might be concerned that common physical problems indicate the cancer is progressing if you have metastatic breast cancer. However, keep in mind that not all changes indicate a worsening of breast cancer. For instance, weariness is frequently seen as a sign of metastatic cancer. Additionally, it is a side effect of widely used cancer treatments, including radiation and chemotherapy. Having said that, don't be afraid to consult your doctor if you consistently feel worn out, lack appetite, or discover that you're losing weight on autopilot.

Other particular symptoms could indicate metastatic breast cancer. These signs vary according to the cancer's spread   location:

Bones

abrupt discomfort in the bones or joints. bones that shatter or fracture more frequently. Your arms and legs may feel numb or weak. Growing.

Mind

headaches or head pressure getting worse. problems such as bright flashes, double vision, or blurry vision.

seizures.

vomiting as well as nausea.
Alterations in behavior or personality.
lungs

A persistent cough.
Dyspnea is an inability to breathe.
ache in the chest.
repeated infections in the chest.
Jaundice of the liver.
rash or skin irritation.
nausea, vomiting, loss of appetite, and stomach pain

Why does breast cancer metastasize?
Recurrent breast cancer, which is defined as cancer that returned following therapy and is now impacting tissue and organs distant from the original breast cancer tumor, accounts for the majority of metastatic breast cancer cases. Nevertheless, 6% of women and individuals with AFAB backgrounds who are diagnosed with breast cancer already have metastatic breast cancer. When treatment fails to completely eradicate cancer cells, breast cancer usually returns. Tumors can be reduced by treatments to the point where they are not

visible on testing. Not all cancerous tumor removal surgeries are 100% successful. Prior to surgery, cancer cells may invade surrounding tissue, lymph nodes, or the bloodstream.

After therapy, these cancer cells may still be present in your body. The cells become stronger over time. They begin to spread and flourish once more. Through your circulation and lymphatic system, these cells may spread cancer to other parts of your body by utilizing your blood vessels and lymph nodes. Breast cancer cells can easily spread throughout your body and find new locations to settle and form tumors, thanks to the fluid carried by your lymph nodes and blood vessels. Breast cancer cells may begin generating new tumors immediately, leading to symptoms or indicators that the cancer has progressed over time. Sometimes, for months or years following therapy, they lie dormant, which means they're not developing or spreading. This is one of the reasons why metastatic breast cancer might manifest years after the conclusion of treatment.

Diagnoses and examinations

How is breast cancer that has spread detected?

In the event that you exhibit signs of metastatic breast cancer, your physician might suggest the following tests: A biopsy is the removal of a sample of tissue for microscopic examination by a medical pathologist. blood tests, such as a full metabolic panel and a complete blood count. If there is a suspicious area in your lungs, you may need a bronchoscopy, which is a procedure that looks within your lungs using a scope. Imaging examinations include CT, MRI, PET, ultrasound, bone scans, and chest X-rays. "Taps" to drain fluid from symptom-affected areas. A pleural tap, for instance, eliminates fluid from the lung region. Fluid from the spinal cord region is removed via a spinal tap. Handling and medical interventions How is breast cancer that has spread treated? As of right now, metastatic breast cancer is incurable. Healthcare professionals concentrate on therapies that help patients live as long as possible with the highest quality of life and the fewest adverse effects. Therefore, there isn't a single treatment for metastatic breast cancer. Treatment plans are created by providers using criteria such as:

kind of breast cancer. When treating metastatic triple-negative breast cancer, medical professionals treat it differently from other, more prevalent forms of the disease, like hormone-positive breast cancer. where the spread of cancer has occurred. For instance, the treatment for breast cancer in the lungs can differ from that for breast cancer in the liver.

previous therapy for breast cancer. Providers take into account how you were affected by treatment and how the cancer responded to it. outcomes of a lab test. Under a microscope, medical pathologists inspect cancer cells to observe their appearance and behavior. What specific therapies are available for breast cancer that has spread? chemotherapy.

hormone   treatment.

immunotherapy.

focused   treatment.

What   is   the   duration   of   treatment?

Should you have undergone treatment for early-stage

breast cancer, you might be acquainted with regimens

that entail administering cancer medications over a

certain duration. Then, getting rid of cancer was the aim.

Currently, the objectives are to lessen the size of newly

formed tumors, stop the cancer from spreading, and

assist you in managing your symptoms. This implies that

your   course   of   treatment   could   last   forever.

**Do medical professionals use surgery to treat
metastatic   breast   cancer?**

Since metastatic breast cancer frequently spreads to

multiple sites, medical professionals usually do not

advise surgery. They might advise surgery to relieve

particular symptoms. For instance, if your liver is

affected by breast cancer, surgery may be necessary to

remove tumors preventing your liver from functioning

properly.

Prevention

Is it possible to stop breast cancer from spreading? Sadly, there is no method to stop the spread of breast cancer. It is crucial to keep in mind that metastatic breast cancer is not caused by your actions or inactions. Because some malignant cells in your breast survived therapy and moved through your lymphatic or circulatory systems, you run the risk of developing metastatic breast cancer. How may my risk be reduced? Monitoring your general health and keeping a lookout for any possible symptoms of metastatic cancer is one strategy to reduce your risk. Treatment can impede the spread of metastatic cancer, but it cannot stop it.

Prognosis and Outlook

What should I anticipate if my breast cancer has spread?

You will schedule routine follow-up appointments with your healthcare practitioner if you are receiving treatment. In addition to asking you about any new symptoms or concerns, they will assess your general health. To determine whether the treatment is having an impact, tests will be conducted.

What is the survival rate of breast cancer with metastases?

Five years after diagnosis, 1 in 3 women and adults with AFAB were still living, according to the U.S. National Cancer Institute. Try to keep in mind that survival rates are only estimations when considering them. How long someone will live with metastatic breast cancer is not indicated by a survival rate. It's also critical to keep in mind that a variety of factors, including your general health, the type of breast cancer you have, and any prior therapies, may have an impact on your circumstances. Speak with your healthcare practitioner if you have any questions concerning the survival statistics of metastatic breast cancer. They are your greatest source of knowledge on what to expect because they are familiar with you.

How does one manage to live with breast cancer that has spread?

Living with metastatic breast cancer might be quite similar in certain aspects. You're still attempting to manage your symptoms, getting therapy, and adjusting to the day-to-day difficulties brought on by a serious disease. The distinction is that you have cancer in several regions of your body, and it is unlikely to get better. Hearing that news is probably very difficult. It could make you feel powerless or like you've lost all control over your life. If that describes your circumstances, you can take the following actions to help manage stress in your particular situation: Think about palliative care for breast cancer that has spread. Palliative care experts assist you in managing symptoms and adverse effects of treatment. Furthermore, palliative care provides tools to support you in managing your mental health. Consume the healthiest diet possible. Your appetite may change as a result of treatment. Ask to consult with a dietitian if you're worried about your diet.

They will offer recommendations for foods. Go easy on yourself. Living with metastatic breast cancer can make one feel as though they are competing in an endless race. Try your best to move more slowly and cautiously.

When should I visit my medical professional?
If you observe any changes in a new location of your body that can indicate breast cancer, get in touch with your provider.

What inquiries ought I make of my healthcare professional?

If your doctor has diagnosed you with metastatic breast cancer, find out:

What alternatives do I have for treatment?

Which way do I stand?

What adverse effects should I anticipate?

Will receiving supplemental therapy improve my condition?

How may I end treatment if I so choose?

How can I get the most out of my treatment?

Other Frequently Asked Questions

Does breast cancer with metastases go into remission?

Depending on the type of breast cancer, the answer may vary. One study, for instance, showed cases where treatment resulted in a nine-year remission of metastatic HER2-positive breast cancer. Remission is the state in which testing reveals no evidence of cancer and you are symptom-free. The phrase "no evidence of disease" may be used by medical professionals. Your medical team will discuss whether your kind of breast cancer is likely to go into remission after spreading if you are undergoing treatment for metastatic breast cancer.

What occurs if I choose to discontinue my treatment? Treatment for metastatic breast cancer includes goal-setting. It's possible that you want to stick with your treatment, no matter what negative effects there are. However, if you believe that the treatment is lowering your quality of life, you might wish to discontinue it. Still, quitting treatment is a big choice. It's also really private.

Find out from your medical team what to anticipate from your therapy if you're thinking about setting goals for it.

Spend some time explaining your decision to discontinue treatment to the people you care about. Moreover, be aware that quitting treatment does not imply ending care. Your medical staff will be by your side, prepared to assist you in every way they can.

Conclusion.

In most parts of the world, breast cancer is the most frequent type of malignancy in women. While HPV has stabilized in Western nations, other continents are seeing an increase in its prevalence. Because the causes of breast cancer are not well understood, prevention is challenging.

Unchecked cell development is cancer. Gene mutations have the potential to accelerate the pace of cell division or prevent the body from regulating regular processes like cell cycle arrest or programmed cell death, which can lead to cancer. A mass of malignant cells has the potential to grow into a tumor. According to the report, 46.36% of people have an overall lack of information about breast cancer. The participants' awareness and practice of breast self-examination and screening techniques were lacking, but their understanding of risk factors, indicators, and symptoms was ordinary.